Sinusitis Diet and Cookbook

A Comprehensive Guide to Managing Sinusitis and Improving Quality of Life.

Title:
Sinusitis Diet and Cookbook

Subtitle

A Comprehensive Guide to Managing Sinusitis and Improving Quality of Life.

Copyright © 2024 by (Dr. Joey Green)

Printed in the United States of America.

ISBN: 9798882881312

TABLE OF CONTENT

INTRODUCTION

Sinusitis is a widespread ailment that affects millions of individuals all over the world. It is characterized by a wide range of symptoms, including irritation, pain, and other symptoms. If you want to be able to properly manage sinusitis, it is very necessary to have a complete awareness of the illness as well as the numerous elements that might contribute to the formation and increase of the condition. In this introductory section, we will dig into the complexities of sinusitis, examining its causes, symptoms, and the consequences it has for one's general health. As an additional topic of discussion, we will investigate the crucial part that nutrition plays in the management of sinusitis, as well as how alterations to one's diet

can ease symptoms and promote sinus health.

Understanding Sinusitis

A swelling or inflammation of the tissue lining the sinuses is called sinusitis, or rhinosinusitis. The main job of the air-filled sinuses, which are found in the bones surrounding the nose and eyes, is to produce mucus, which helps to moisten the air we breathe and traps germs, pollutants, and other particles before they enter the lungs.

Mucus cannot adequately drain from the sinus passages when they are inflamed or obstructed, whether from an infection, allergies, or other conditions. This causes a build-up of fluid and pressure. Symptoms include face discomfort, pressure, congestion, nasal discharge, coughing, and diminished taste and smell perception can result from this accumulation.

Based on the length and intensity of symptoms, sinusitis can be divided into many types:

- Acute Sinusitis: Transient inflammation of the sinuses, frequently brought on by a cold or other viral illness. Less than four weeks is the average duration of symptoms, which can go away on their own or with therapy.

- Subacute Sinusitis: An inflammation that lasts four to twelve weeks. It usually happens after an acute sinus infection, although it can also be brought on by a chronic allergy or irritation.

- Chronic Sinusitis: An inflammation that lasts for 12 weeks or more and may not go away with therapy. Underlying illnesses including nasal polyps, a deviated septum, or immune system problems might result in chronic sinusitis.

- Recurrent Sinusitis: Several bouts of acute sinusitis spaced a year apart by intervals during which the symptoms subside.

Effective management and treatment of sinusitis require an understanding of the condition's kind and underlying cause. Acute sinusitis frequently goes away on its own or with little treatment, while chronic or recurring sinusitis may need more involved management techniques, such as dietary changes.

Importance of Diet in Managing Sinusitis

Due to its effects on inflammation, immunological response, and general sinus health, diet is an important management strategy for sinusitis. While certain foods have anti-inflammatory and immune-boosting qualities that can help reduce symptoms and encourage recovery, others might increase nasal congestion and inflammation.

The following are the main arguments in favor of nutrition in sinusitis management:

- Control of Inflammation: One of the main characteristics of sinusitis is persistent inflammation. Certain eating habits, such as eating a lot of processed foods, refined carbohydrates, and unhealthy fats, can cause inflammation in the nasal passages and other parts of the body. On the other hand, a diet high in fruits, vegetables, whole grains, and healthy fats can aid in lowering inflammation and relieving sinusitis symptoms.

- Immune Support: Repelling infections and preserving sinus health depend on a robust immune system. Meals strong in zinc, selenium, and vitamins A, C, and E are examples of nutrient-rich foods that can boost immunity and help prevent sinus infections from happening again. Furthermore, foods high in probiotics, including kefir, yogurt, and fermented veggies, help support a balanced population of gut bacteria, which is essential for immunological control.

- Mucus Production: Drinking enough water and eating specific meals might help thin mucus secretions, which facilitates nasal drainage and relieves congestion. Mucus may be kept flowing and sinus pressure can be reduced by consuming hydrating meals such as soups, broths, and herbal teas along with drinking enough water throughout the day.

- Management of Allergies: Dietary variables can either increase or alleviate allergy symptoms. Allergies are a major cause of sinusitis. For those who suffer from allergic sinusitis, recognizing and eliminating certain dietary allergens, such as dairy, gluten, and artificial additives, can help lessen swelling and congestion.

- General Health: Eating a well-balanced and nourishing diet helps to maintain nasal health as well as general health. People can improve their health and lower their chance of developing chronic illnesses that could worsen sinusitis by emphasizing full, nutrient-dense diets and reducing their intake of processed and inflammatory carbohydrates.

WHAT IS SINUSITIS?

The common medical condition known as sinusitis, also called rhinosinusitis or sinus infection, is characterized by swelling or inflammation of the tissue lining the sinuses. The sinuses, which are hollow cavities found in the bones surrounding the nose and eyes, are essential for the production of mucus, which purges pollutants, allergens, and particles from the air and traps them. The mucus cannot adequately drain from irritated or clogged sinuses, which causes a fluid and pressure buildup. This accumulation can result in a variety of symptoms, from moderate soreness to excruciating pain and congestion.

Types of Sinusitis

Depending on the length and intensity of symptoms, there are many forms of sinusitis:

1. Acute Sinusitis: Typically brought on by a viral illness like the flu or the common cold, acute sinusitis is a transient inflammation of the sinuses. Additionally, fungal growth or bacterial infections in the sinuses may be the cause. The symptoms of acute sinusitis may appear suddenly and include nasal congestion, face discomfort or pressure, thick, colorful nasal discharge, coughing, exhaustion, and diminished taste and smell perception. Less than four weeks is the

typical duration of symptoms, which can go away on their own or with therapy.

2. Subacute Sinusitis: This type of inflammation lasts for four to twelve weeks. It frequently arises as a consequence of a recurring allergy or irritation, or it follows an acute sinus infection. Similar to acute sinusitis, subacute sinusitis might have more extended or severe symptoms.

3. Chronic Sinusitis: Despite therapeutic efforts, chronic sinusitis is typified by inflammation that lasts for 12 weeks or more. It might be the consequence of underlying illnesses including immune system problems, deviated septums, or

nasal polyps. Chronic sinusitis can cause nasal congestion that doesn't go away, pressure or pain in the face, nasal discharge, coughing, headaches, exhaustion, and diminished taste and smell perception. The quality of life can be greatly impacted by chronic sinusitis, which may call for more involved management techniques such as medication, nasal irrigation, and even surgery.

4. Recurrent Sinusitis: This condition is defined as several acute sinusitis episodes that occur within a year, interspersed with times when the symptoms subside. People who have recurrent sinusitis may get acute sinus

infections, which are frequently brought on by allergies, bacterial or viral pathogens, or environmental irritants. Effectively treating symptoms and avoiding recurring sinus infections depend on identifying and resolving underlying causes.

Causes and Symptoms

Numerous causes, like as infections, allergies, structural irregularities, and environmental irritants, might contribute to the development of sinusitis. Effective management and treatment of sinusitis depend on an understanding of its underlying causes.

1. Infections: The most frequent cause of acute sinusitis is a viral infection, such as the common cold or influenza. Congestion, mucus accumulation, and sinus pressure might result from these illnesses' ability to inflame and expand the sinus linings. Infections with bacteria can also happen on their own or as a side effect of viral

infections, especially in situations of acute or persistent sinusitis. Fungal infections are also possible, although they are less frequent and usually affect those with compromised immune systems or underlying medical issues.

2. Allergies: Another important cause of sinusitis is allergic rhinitis, sometimes referred to as hay fever. Allergies to airborne particles like mold, dust mites, pollen, or pet dander can inflame the sinuses and nasal passages, resulting in symptoms including sinus pressure, sneezing, congestion, and itching. In addition to common allergy symptoms including itchy eyes, sore throats,

and skin rashes, allergic sinusitis frequently manifests as a clear nasal discharge.

3. Structural Abnormalities: Deviated septa, nasal polyps, and sinus cysts are examples of structural abnormalities of the nasal passages or sinuses that can impede normal sinus drainage and ventilation, making people more susceptible to chronic sinusitis and recurrent sinus infections. These anomalies can range in severity from moderate to major and can be either congenital or acquired.

4. Environmental Irritants: The sinus linings can become irritated and more inflamed by exposure to environmental irritants such as

cigarette smoke, air pollution, harsh smells, and chemical fumes. This can result in the symptoms of sinusitis. People who work in settings with high concentrations of allergens or air pollution may be more prone to sinusitis.

Symptoms of Sinusitis

Depending on the kind, intensity, and underlying cause of the illness, sinusitis can have a variety of symptoms. Typical sinusitis symptoms include:

- Stuffiness or congestion of the nose.
- Cough; might be more severe at night.
- Diminished taste and smell perception.
- Ears fullness or pressure.
- Headache, especially in the temples or forehead.
- Toothache, particularly in the front teeth.
- Weariness and sultry mood.
- Facial pressure or discomfort, especially in the areas surrounding the eyes, cheeks, and forehead.

- Thick secretions from the nose, frequently green or yellow in hue.

- Dripping from the nose (mucus dripping down the back of the throat).

In contrast to chronic sinusitis, which causes symptoms that may become more persistent or recurring over time, acute sinusitis symptoms usually appear unexpectedly and may be severe. A medical professional's consultation is necessary for a precise diagnosis and suitable treatment of sinusitis, as certain symptoms may mimic those of other ailments including allergies, migraines, or dental issues.

HOW DIET AFFECTS SINUSITIS

Due to its ability to either worsen or lessen inflammation, congestion, and other symptoms related to sinusitis, diet is important in controlling the illness. While certain foods have anti-inflammatory and immune-boosting qualities that can help reduce symptoms and support sinus health, others might cause the body to respond inflammatory, increasing sinus congestion and pain. This section will discuss how nutrition might impact sinusitis, including foods that exacerbate symptoms and those that alleviate them.

Foods that Aggravate Sinusitis

Dairy Items: Milk, cheese, and yogurt are examples of dairy products that are frequently linked to increased mucus production and congestion in certain people. Many people claim that their sinus pressure and congestion worsen after ingesting dairy, even though scientific information on the subject is conflicting. This might be because dairy products include lactose or other substances that, in sensitive people, can increase mucus production or cause inflammation.

- Refined Sugars: Consuming foods high in refined sugars, such as sweets, sugary snacks, and sweetened beverages, can weaken the immune system and cause inflammation, which may exacerbate sinusitis symptoms. Consuming a lot of sugar has been related to oxidative stress and increased inflammatory cytokine production in the body, both of which can aggravate sinus congestion and inflammation.

- Fast food, packaged snacks, and ready-to-eat meals are examples of processed foods. These foods frequently include high amounts of salt, artificial additives, and unhealthy fats, all of which can exacerbate sinusitis symptoms and cause inflammation. These foods may damage gut health, which can affect immune function and worsen inflammation throughout the body, including the sinuses, because they are often poor in nutrients and fiber.

- Spicy Foods: For some people, spicy foods like hot peppers, chili peppers, and spicy sauces can aggravate sinus congestion and inflammation by irritating the nasal passages. The main ingredient in peppers that gives them their heat, capsaicin, can cause sinus and nasal congestion and burning in the nose. It can also cause mucus production to rise.

- Alcohol: Because alcohol dehydrates the body and can aggravate nasal congestion and inflammation, it can make sinusitis symptoms worse. In addition to impairing immune system function and sleep habits, alcohol can increase an individual's susceptibility to sinus infections and exacerbations.

- Caffeine: While most people believe moderate caffeine intake to be acceptable, consuming large amounts of caffeinated beverages—such as energy drinks, tea, and coffee—can increase sinus pressure and dehydrate people. Due to its diuretic properties, caffeine can cause fluid loss and increased urine output, which can aggravate symptoms of dehydration and nose dryness.

- Foods High in Sodium: Foods high in sodium, such as canned soups, processed meats, and salty snacks, can exacerbate nasal swelling and fluid retention. Consuming too much salt can raise blood pressure and cause fluid to accumulate in the body, especially in the sinuses, which can make sinusitis symptoms worse.

Foods that Alleviate Sinusitis

- Anti-inflammatory Foods: You can lessen inflammation and the symptoms of sinusitis by including anti-inflammatory foods in your diet. These include leafy greens, berries, citrus fruits, and cruciferous vegetables like Brussels sprouts and broccoli. They also include fruits and vegetables high in phytochemicals and antioxidants. Walnuts, flaxseeds, and fatty fish are good sources of omega-3 fatty acids, which can also help lower inflammation and improve sinus health.

- Foods That Will Hydrate You: It's important to drink plenty of water to thin mucus secretions and encourage healthy sinus drainage. Eating foods high in water content, such as oranges, cucumbers, and watermelon, as well as hydrating soups, broths, and herbal teas can help keep the nasal passages moist and reduce congestion. In addition to avoiding excessive coffee and alcohol usage, which can exacerbate dehydration, sinus health also requires avoiding these substances.

- Herbs and Spices: A few herbs and spices have decongestant and anti-inflammatory qualities that may help reduce the symptoms of sinusitis. Due to their anti-inflammatory qualities, ginger, turmeric, garlic, and onions can be added to soups, stir-fries, and teas to help lessen congestion and inflammation in the sinuses. When taken in moderation, horseradish, wasabi, and mustard can also aid in sinus drainage and nasal passage clearance.

- Probiotic-Rich Foods: Eating foods high in probiotics, like kefir, kimchi, sauerkraut, and yogurt, can boost immunity and promote gut health, which lowers the risk of sinus infections and flare-ups. Probiotics are made up of good bacteria that support a balanced gut microbiota, which is essential for immune system function and inflammation management. Regularly including foods high in probiotics in your diet can help keep your sinuses healthy and stop recurrent sinusitis.

- Warm and Moist Foods: Eating warm, moist food can aid in sinus drainage and the calming of irritated nasal passages. Herbal teas, steaming veggies, and warm soups can help thin mucus secretions and relieve pressure and congestion in the sinuses. Foods that are cold or frozen should be avoided as they can worsen congestion and discomfort in those who have sinusitis.

- Hydration: Sustaining sinus health and encouraging appropriate mucus production and drainage require adequate hydration.

Throughout the day, sipping lots of water can help thin mucus secretions and avoid dehydration, both of which can make sinusitis symptoms worse. Try to drink eight glasses or more of water each day, and if you suffer from symptoms of dehydration like headaches, dry mouth, or dark urine, up your fluid intake.

CREATING A SINUSITIS-FRIENDLY DIET PLAN

Making dietary decisions that are strategic to minimize inflammation, enhance sinus health, and alleviate symptoms is an important part of managing sinusitis with diet. A diet plan that is suitable for sinusitis places an emphasis on foods that are high in nutrients and aid in the operation of the immune system, reduce inflammation, and encourage appropriate sinus outflow. In this part of the article, we will discuss the fundamentals of a sinusitis diet, which will include the fundamental rules that should be adhered to, as well as some recommendations for meal planning that will assist you in incorporating good eating habits into your daily routine.

Basics of a Sinusitis Diet

Emphasis on Whole Foods: Make fruits, vegetables, whole grains, lean meats, and healthy fats the main components of your diet. Avoid processed foods. These foods are high in fiber, antioxidants, and other vital nutrients that promote immune function, lower inflammation, and improve general health.

Stress Anti-Inflammatory Foods: Include a wide variety of anti-inflammatory foods in your diet, including berries, leafy greens, nuts, seeds, olive oil, and fatty fish (such as salmon, mackerel, and sardines). Antioxidants and omega-3 fatty acids included in these foods aid in the reduction of inflammation and support sinus health.

Reduce Inflammatory Foods: Reducing your consumption of meals high in trans fats, processed foods, refined sweets, and excessive levels of saturated fats can all worsen the symptoms of sinusitis. These foods may exacerbate sinus pain and congestion by increasing inflammation in the body.

Keep Yourself Hydrated: To aid in thinning mucus production and fostering appropriate nasal outflow, sip plenty of water throughout the day. At least eight glasses of water should be consumed each day, and excessive coffee and alcohol use should be avoided since they can worsen the symptoms of sinusitis and cause dehydration.

Mix in Immune-Supporting Foods: Include foods that strengthen the immune system in your diet to help your body's defenses against infections and to maintain the health of your sinuses. Citrus fruits (oranges, lemons, grapefruits), garlic, ginger, turmeric, and foods high in probiotics, such as kefir, sauerkraut, and yogurt, are a few examples.

Use Low-Sodium Alternatives: To assist decrease nasal congestion and reduce fluid retention, select low-sodium alternatives wherever feasible. Reduce the amount of processed foods, canned soups, and salty snacks you consume in favor of handmade or fresh meals that are seasoned with natural flavorings and herbs.

Try Adding Herbs and Spices with Anti-Inflammatory Properties to Your Food: Adding anti-inflammatory herbs and spices to your cooking can enhance its flavor and increase its nutritional value. Ginger, turmeric, garlic, onions, cayenne pepper, cinnamon, and rosemary are a few examples.

Maintain Balance in Your Diet: Although some foods may be good for sinus health, it's important to maintain balance in your diet. To prevent overindulging, consume a range of meals in sensible portion sizes and pay attention to your body's signals of hunger and fullness.

Meal Planning Tips

Plan Ahead: Give your schedule, dietary requirements, and nutritional preferences some thought as you organize your meals and snacks for the next week. Making better food selections and avoiding grabbing fast food or convenience meals when pressed for time is made easier when you follow a meal plan.

Cook in Bulk: Take into consideration preparing meals in bulk and storing them for later use. This can guarantee that you always have wholesome meals available when you need them and can save time and effort during hectic workdays. Grain-based salads, stews, casseroles, and soups are great choices for cooking in large quantities.

Incorporate Variety: To make sure you're receiving a wide range of nutrients and tastes in your meals, try to include a variety of foods from all the food categories. To make your meals interesting and fulfilling, try experimenting with different fruits, veggies, whole grains, proteins, and plant-based fats.

Prepare Ingredients Ahead of Time: To simplify meal preparation and ease cooking throughout the week, wash, cut, and prepare fruits, vegetables, and other ingredients ahead of time. For easy access, store prepared items in the refrigerator in sealed containers.

Stock Up on Nuts, Seeds, Herbs, and Spices: Maintain a supply of healthful grains, canned beans, frozen fruits and veggies, nuts, and seeds in your pantry, refrigerator, and freezer. Keeping these ingredients on hand facilitates quick and easy preparation of wholesome meals and snacks.

Plan for Days When You're Short on Time or Energy: Make sure to include quick and easy meal alternatives in your meal plan for those days. You can quickly produce quick meals like salads, sandwiches, smoothies, and grain bowls and personalize them with your favorite ingredients.

Be Adaptable: Adjust your food plan in response to shifting conditions, inclinations, or desires. To keep your meals interesting and fun, don't be scared to try out new flavors, recipes, and ingredients.

Pay Attention to Your Body: Observe your reactions to various meals and modify your diet accordingly. If you find that particular foods make your sinusitis symptoms worse, you should think about removing or cutting them from your diet in favor of meals that provide you with energy and nourishment.

ESSENTIAL NUTRIENTS FOR SINUS HEALTH

One of the most important things for one's general health and quality of life is to keep their sinuses in good condition. There is a significant contribution that nutrients make to the maintenance of immunological function, the reduction of inflammation, and the promotion of healthy sinus drainage and function. The necessary elements for sinus health, such as vitamins, minerals, antioxidants, and foods that reduce inflammation, will be discussed in this portion of the book.

Vitamins and Minerals

- Vitamin C: An effective antioxidant, vitamin C is essential for boosting the immune system and lowering inflammation. It contributes to the immune system's strengthening, increasing its resistance to infections, especially sinus infections. Citrus fruits (including oranges, lemons, and grapefruits), strawberries, kiwis, bell peppers, broccoli, and Brussels sprouts are foods high in vitamin C.

- Vitamin A: The mucous membranes lining the respiratory tract, especially the sinuses, depend on vitamin A to be healthy. It helps guard against irritants and infections by maintaining the integrity of the epithelial cells lining the sinus passages. Vitamin A-rich foods include liver, cantaloupe, spinach, kale, sweet potatoes, and carrots.

- Vitamin E: Rich in antioxidant properties, vitamin E helps shield cells from inflammation and oxidative stress. It enhances immunological response and could lessen sinusitis symptoms. Almonds, sunflower seeds, hazelnuts, spinach, avocado, and wheat germ are among the foods high in vitamin E.

- Zinc: An important mineral, zinc is necessary for both wound healing and immune system function. It may lessen the length and intensity of sinus infections and aid in immune cell activity. Oysters, cattle, pigs, poultry, lentils, chickpeas, and pumpkin seeds are among the foods high in zinc.

- Selenium: This trace element supports immune system function and functions as an antioxidant. It may help lessen nasal irritation and shield cells from oxidative damage. Selenium-rich foods include eggs, sunflower seeds, seafood (including tuna, shrimp, and sardines), Brazil nuts, and sunflower seeds.

- Magnesium: The body uses magnesium for approximately 300 metabolic processes, including immune system response and muscle relaxation. It could lessen headaches and tense muscles that are brought on by sinusitis. Dark chocolate, whole grains, legumes, nuts, seeds, and leafy green vegetables are among the foods high in magnesium.

- Potassium: Potassium is a necessary mineral that controls neuron activity, muscular contractions, and fluid balance. It could support the body's normal electrolyte balance and hydration, both of which are critical for sinus health. Salmon, sweet potatoes, avocado, bananas, spinach, and yogurt are among the foods high in potassium.

Antioxidants and Anti-inflammatory Foods

Berries: Antioxidants known as flavonoids, which have immune-stimulating and anti-inflammatory qualities, are abundant in berries including blueberries, strawberries, raspberries, and blackberries. They aid in reducing inflammation in many parts of the body, including the sinuses, and neutralizing free radicals.

Leafy Green Vegetables: Rich in vitamins, minerals, and antioxidants that boost the immune system and lower inflammation are leafy greens including spinach, kale, Swiss chard, and collard greens. They also include fiber, which supports sinus health indirectly and aids in the promotion of gut health.

Cruciferous Vegetables: Containing sulfur compounds and antioxidants, cruciferous vegetables like broccoli, Brussels sprouts, cabbage, and cauliflower aid in the body's detoxification processes and decrease inflammation. Additionally, they include vitamins and minerals that are critical for a healthy immune system and general well-being.

Curcumin, a substance found in turmeric, is a spice with strong anti-inflammatory and antioxidant qualities. It may lessen sinusitis symptoms and aid in the body's reduction of inflammation. Because of its health advantages, turmeric may be added to smoothies, drinks, curries, and soups.

Another spice that can reduce inflammation and strengthen the immune system is ginger. It helps control the symptoms of sinusitis by reducing inflammation in the respiratory system and sinuses. Ginger may be used in baking, cooking, and drinks either fresh or dried or powdered.

Garlic and Onions: Packed with antioxidants and sulfur compounds, garlic and onions aid in immunological support, inflammation reduction, and sinus health. Additionally, they include antibacterial qualities that might aid in the fight against respiratory tract and sinus infections.

Fatty Fish: Omega-3 fatty acids, which have anti-inflammatory qualities, are abundant in fatty fish, including trout, sardines, salmon, and mackerel. They boost immune system activity and aid in reducing inflammation all across the body, including the sinuses. Frequent consumption of fatty fish may help lessen sinusitis symptoms and lower the chance of infection.

RECIPES FOR SINUSITIS RELIEF

Through the management of sinusitis, the incorporation of foods that are abundant in nutrients and possess anti-inflammatory characteristics can assist in the alleviation of symptoms and the promotion of sinus health. In this area, we will discuss several different recipes that are intended to alleviate the symptoms of sinusitis. Known for their ability to strengthen the immune system, reduce inflammation, and clear sinuses, the ingredients that are featured in these recipes are the center of attention.

5 Breakfast Ideas

Turmeric Golden Milk Smoothie:

Ingredients:

- One ripe banana.

- a cup of almond milk without sugar (or any milk of choice).

- Half a teaspoon of turmeric powder.

- 1/4 tsp ground ginger.

- 1/4 tsp ground cinnamon.

- One spoonful of maple syrup or honey (optional).

- Half a teaspoon of extract from vanilla beans.

- A little amount of black pepper (to enhance turmeric absorption).

Instructions:

- Put all the ingredients in a blender and process until smooth.
- Enjoy the smoothie right away after pouring it into a glass.

Berry Spinach Smoothie:

Ingredients:

- 1 cup mixed berries, either fresh or frozen (such as strawberries, blueberries, and raspberries).
- A single handful of young spinach leaves.
- 1/2 cup Greek yogurt, plain.
- One spoonful of maple syrup or honey (optional).
- 1/2 cup almond milk, unsweetened (or any milk of choice).

Instructions:

- Put all the ingredients in a blender and process until smooth.

- If extra milk is required to get the right consistency, add it.

- Enjoy the smoothie after pouring it into a glass.

Avocado Toast with Poached Egg:

Ingredients:

- Two toasted whole-grain pieces of bread.

- Mash one ripe avocado.

- two eggs.

- To taste, add salt and pepper.

- Flakes of red pepper (optional).

Instructions:

- For around three to four minutes, or until the whites are set but the yolks are still runny, poach the eggs in boiling water.

- Evenly distribute the avocado mash over the slices of toasted bread.

- Place a poached egg on top of each piece.

- If preferred, add red pepper flakes, salt, and pepper for seasoning.

- Serve right away.

Oatmeal with Berries and Almonds:

Ingredients:

- Half a cup of rolled oats.

- One cup of water or your preferred milk.

- Half a cup of mixed berries (such as strawberries, blueberries, and raspberries).

- Almonds, cut, two tablespoons.

- One spoonful of maple syrup or honey (optional).

- A little amount of ground cinnamon.

Instructions:

- Heat the milk or water in a saucepan until it begins to boil.

- After adding the rolled oats, turn down the heat. Cook for 5 to 7 minutes, stirring often, or until the oats are soft.

- After turning off the heat, scoop the oats into a bowl.

- Add sliced almonds, honey, or maple syrup (if using), mixed berries, and a dash of cinnamon on top.

- Warm-up and savor.

Greek Yogurt Parfait:

Ingredients:

- One cup of Greek yogurt, plain.

- Half a cup of granola.

- Half a cup of mixed berries (such as strawberries, blueberries, and raspberries).

- One spoonful of maple syrup or honey (optional).

Instructions:

- Arrange the Greek yogurt, granola, and mixed berries in a glass or dish.

- If desired, drizzle with maple syrup or honey.

- Until the glass or bowl is filled, keep adding layers.

- Serve right away as a filling and healthy breakfast choice.

5 Lunch and Dinner Recipes

Chicken and Vegetable Stir-Fry:

Ingredients:

- Two skinless, boneless chicken breasts, cut thinly.
- Two cups of mixed veggies (such as bell peppers, broccoli, carrots, and snap peas).
- two minced garlic cloves.
- One tablespoon of freshly grated ginger.
- Two teaspoons of soy sauce reduced in sodium.
- One tablespoon of sesame oil.
- Prepared quinoa or brown rice for serving.

Instructions:

- In a large skillet or wok, heat the sesame oil over medium-high heat.

- Add the chicken slices and heat for 5 to 7 minutes, or until browned and cooked through.

- Cook for an additional minute after adding the grated ginger and minced garlic to the skillet.

- Stir-fry the mixed veggies in the pan with the soy sauce for three to five minutes, or until the vegetables are crisp-tender.

- Serve the stir-fry over quinoa or cooked brown rice.

Salmon with Roasted Vegetables:

Ingredients:

- Two fillets of salmon.

- Two cups of mixed veggies (such as asparagus, bell peppers, zucchini, and cherry tomatoes).

- Two teaspoons of olive oil.

- two minced garlic cloves.

- One tsp of dried thyme.

- To taste, add salt and pepper.

Instructions:

- Set oven temperature to 400°F, or 200°C.

- Arrange the salmon fillets onto a parchment paper-lined baking sheet.

- Combine the mixed veggies in a bowl with the olive oil, dried thyme, minced garlic, salt, and pepper.

- Arrange the salmon on the baking sheet with the seasoned veggies surrounding it.

- Roast for 15 to 20 minutes in a preheated oven, or until the veggies are soft and the salmon is well cooked.

- Warm up the roasted veggies and fish.

Quinoa Salad with Chickpeas and Lemon Vinaigrette:

Ingredients:

- 1 cup of quinoa, cooked.

- One 15-oz can of washed and drained chickpeas.

- One chopped cucumber.

- One sliced bell pepper.

- 1/4 cup of finely sliced red onion.

- 1/4 cup finely chopped fresh parsley.

- One lemon juice.

- Two teaspoons of olive oil.

- To taste, add salt and pepper.

Instructions:

- The cooked quinoa, chickpeas, sliced cucumber, bell pepper, red onion, and chopped parsley should all be combined in a big bowl.

- To create the vinaigrette, combine the lemon juice, olive oil, salt, and pepper in a small bowl.

- After adding the vinaigrette, mix the quinoa salad to ensure uniform coating.

- The salad can be served cold or at room temperature.

Vegetable and Lentil Soup:

Ingredients:

- One tablespoon of extra virgin olive oil.

- One sliced onion.

- two minced garlic cloves.

- Diced two carrots.

- Diced two celery stalks.

- Rinse and drain 1 cup of dry green lentils.

- Six glasses of broth made with vegetables.

- One tsp of dried thyme.

- One bay leaf.

- To taste, add salt and pepper.

- For a garnish, use fresh parsley (optional).

Instructions:

- In a big saucepan, warm up the olive oil over medium heat.

- Simmer the chopped onion and minced garlic for five minutes, or until the ingredients are tender.

- To the saucepan, add the chopped carrots, celery, green lentils, dried thyme, bay leaf, salt, and pepper.

- After bringing the soup to a boil, lower the heat, cover it, and simmer it for 20 to 25 minutes, or until the veggies and lentils are soft.

- Take out and dispose of the bay leaf from the soup.

- If preferred, top the hot soup with some fresh parsley.

Roasted Butternut Squash and Apple Salad:

Ingredients:

- 4 cups of diced butternut squash.

- Two cored and sliced apples.

- Two teaspoons olive oil.

- One tablespoon maple syrup.

- One teaspoon of ground cinnamon.

- 1/4 teaspoon ground nutmeg.

- 4 cups mixed salad greens (such as spinach, arugula, and kale).

- 1/4 cup dried cranberries.

- 1/4 cup chopped pecans.

- Balsamic vinaigrette for dressing.

Instructions:

- Set oven temperature to 400°F, or 200°C.

- Toss the chopped apples and cubed butternut squash with maple syrup, nutmeg, cinnamon, and olive oil in a big bowl until well combined.

- Arrange the seasoned apples and squash in a single layer on a parchment paper-lined baking sheet.

- Roast the squash for 25 to 30 minutes in a preheated oven, or until it's soft and has a light caramelized color.

- Toss the roasted apples and butternut squash with the chopped nuts, dried cranberries, and mixed salad greens in a large salad dish.

- For even coating, drizzle with balsamic vinaigrette and toss.

- Present the salad as a tasty and wholesome choice for lunch or dinner.

5 Snacks and Beverages

Homemade Hummus with Veggie Sticks:

Ingredients:

- One 15-oz can of washed and drained chickpeas.

- Twice as much tahini.

- Two tsp lemon juice.

- One minced garlic clove.

- Two teaspoons of olive oil.

- To taste, add salt and pepper.

- A variety of vegetable sticks for serving, including bell peppers, celery, cucumbers, and carrots.

Instructions:

- Add the chickpeas, tahini, lemon juice, olive oil, minced garlic, salt, and pepper to a food processor.

- If necessary, add a splash of water to get the required consistency after blending until smooth and creamy.

- Move the hummus into a serving bowl and present it alongside a variety of veggie sticks for dunks.

Greek Yogurt with Honey and Walnuts:

Ingredients:

- One cup of Greek yogurt, plain.

- One spoonful of honey.

- Two tablespoons of walnuts chopped.

Instructions:

- Spoon the plain Greek yogurt into a small bowl.

- After adding a honey drizzle, top with chopped walnuts.

- act as a filling and healthy snack choice.

Green Smoothie:

Ingredients:

- 1 cup fresh spinach leaves.

- A half-ripe banana.

- 1/2 cup of pieces of frozen pineapple.

- 1/2 cup almond milk, unsweetened (or any milk of choice).

- One-third cup chia seeds.

- One teaspoon of maple syrup or honey (optional).

Instructions:

- Put all the ingredients in a blender and process until smooth.

- If extra almond milk is required to get the right consistency, add it.

- Enjoy the smoothie after pouring it into a glass.

Turmeric Ginger Tea:

Ingredients:

- 1 teaspoon grated fresh ginger.

- Half a teaspoon of turmeric powder.

- One spoonful of honey.

- Juice from half a lemon.

- One cup of steaming water.

Instructions:

- Grated ginger, powdered turmeric, honey, and lemon juice should all be combined in a cup.

- After adding hot water to the mixture, whisk everything together thoroughly.

- Before sipping, let the tea simmer for a few minutes.

- Savor the warming and calming taste of the turmeric ginger tea.

Vegetable Sushi Rolls:

Ingredients:

- Two sheets of nori seaweed.

- one cup of sushi rice, cooked.

- different sliced veggies (such as cucumber, avocado, carrot, bell pepper, and radish).

- For dipping, use tamari or soy sauce.

- Pickled wasabi with ginger (optional).

Instructions:

- Arrange a sheet of nori seaweed, shiny side down, on a spotless kitchen towel or bamboo sushi mat.

- Leaving a 1-inch margin at the top, evenly distribute half of the cooked sushi rice over the nori sheet.

- Across the middle of the rice, arrange the sliced veggies in a single layer.

- Using a kitchen towel or bamboo sushi mat to assist shape the roll, tightly wrap up the nori sheet starting from the bottom.

- Continue with the remaining ingredients and the nori sheet.

- Cut each sushi roll into bite-sized pieces using a sharp knife.

- Present the veggie sushi rolls with wasabi and pickled ginger on the side, and either soy sauce or tamari for dipping.

COOKING TECHNIQUES FOR SINUSITIS-FRIENDLY MEALS

When it comes to producing sinusitis-friendly meals that are tasty, nutritious, and supportive of sinus health, cooking techniques play a crucial part in the development of these dishes. Enhancing the flavor of your food while simultaneously lowering inflammation and supporting sinus health may be accomplished by concentrating on cooking with a low salt content and employing a wide range of spice and herb combinations. In the following part, we will discuss cooking methods that are advantageous for those who suffer from sinusitis. These methods include cooking with reduced salt levels and coming up with inventive ways to employ culinary herbs and spices.

Low-Sodium Cooking

For those who have sinusitis, lowering sodium consumption is crucial since too much salt can exacerbate nasal swelling and congestion as well as fluid retention. The following advice will help you prepare meals using low-sodium cooking methods:

- Limit Salt: Whenever feasible, cut back on or completely remove additional salt from your recipes. To give your food more depth and complexity, try adding herbs, spices, vinegar, citrus juices, and other flavor-enhancing substances in place of salt.

- Examine the labels: Processed and packaged foods should be avoided since they frequently have high salt content. Whenever feasible, go for low- or no-sodium options; furthermore, choose fresh, whole foods over processed ones.

- Use Fresh Ingredients: To improve taste without adding more salt, add fresh fruits, vegetables, herbs, and spices to your meals. Fresh ingredients may improve the flavor and health of your food by adding natural tastes and nutrients that promote nasal health.

- Homemade Stocks and Broths: Use low-sodium foods like vegetables, herbs, and lean meats to make your stocks and broths. Compared to store-bought equivalents, homemade stocks have less salt and provide you with more control over the flavor and composition of your recipes.

- Herb-Infused Oils and Vinegar: You may flavor your food without adding extra salt by using herb-infused oils and vinegar. Use fresh herbs like garlic, basil, thyme, or rosemary to infuse vinegar or olive oil to make flavorful marinades, sauces, and salads.

- Acidic Components: To lighten tastes and counterbalance richness, add acidic ingredients to your dishes, such as lemon juice, lime juice, balsamic vinegar, and apple cider vinegar. You may use less salt and improve the flavor of your food by using acidic substances.

- Try Different Tasty Spices: To give your food more depth and complexity, experiment with different flavorful spices and spice mixes. Certain spices, such as chili powder, paprika, cumin, and coriander, can offer strong tastes without requiring additional salt.

- Use Fresh Herbs: Adding flavor to your food while cutting down on salt is a great way to use fresh herbs. Try experimenting with different herbs to give your meals more freshness and energy, such as parsley, cilantro, dill, mint, and basil.

Incorporating Herbs and Spices

In addition to giving your food taste and scent, herbs and spices provide several health advantages, such as reducing inflammation and strengthening the immune system. Cooking with herbs and spices may improve the flavor of your food and support healthy sinuses. Use herbs and spices in your meals in these inventive ways:

- Dried vs. Fresh Herbs: Try using both dried and fresh herbs in your cooking. Fresh herbs are best used in salads, dressings, and garnishes since they have a strong flavor and scent and don't need to be cooked much. Since dried herbs have a stronger flavor, they work well in recipes that call for longer cooking durations, such as sauces, stews, and soups.

- Herb Rubs and Marinades: Combine fresh herbs, garlic, zest from citrus, and olive oil to make herb rubs and marinades. To add flavor and moisture to protein, rub the mixture on meat, poultry, or fish before grilling, roasting, or baking.

- Herb-infused Butter: To make herb-infused butter, cut fresh herbs and spices and mix them with melted butter. Toast, muffins, or roasted veggies will all benefit from the taste and richness of the herb butter.

- Spice Blends: Try blending your spices to give your food more nuance and complexity. For flavoring meats, vegetables, grains, and legumes, mix spices like cumin, coriander, turmeric, paprika, and cinnamon to create tasty mixtures.

- Fresh Herb Sauces: To sprinkle over grilled meats, fish, or vegetables, make fresh herb sauces like pesto, chimichurri, or salsa verde. These sauces may be made using various herbs, nuts, and spices to give foods a vibrant, herbaceous taste.

- Herb-infused Oils and Vinegar: To make flavorful oils and vinegar for salad dressing, meat marinating, or bread dipping, infuse olive oil or vinegar with fresh herbs, garlic, or chili peppers. Herb-infused oils and vinegar can be used as a last touch to enhance tastes and give meals depth and complexity.

- Garnishes: To enhance the flavor and aesthetic appeal of your food, garnish it with fresh herbs and spices. For a burst of color and freshness, sprinkle chopped herbs like parsley, cilantro, or chives over salads, soups, pasta dishes, or roasted vegetables.

- Herbal Teas: For a calming and fragrant drink, make herbal teas with fresh or dried herbs like ginger, mint, chamomile, or lemon balm. In addition to being hydrated, herbal teas can reduce inflammation and nasal congestion.

Lifestyle Changes for Managing Sinusitis

Alterations to one's lifestyle, in addition to dietary adjustments and medical therapies, can play a significant role in the management of sinusitis, making it possible to reduce the frequency of symptoms and the severity of their manifestations. Two of the most important aspects of a holistic approach to sinus health are the utilization of stress management strategies and the practice of regular physical activity. In this part of the article, we will discuss the significance of stress management and physical activity in the treatment of sinusitis, as well as offer some suggestions for implementing these lifestyle adjustments into your regularly scheduled activities.

Stress Management

Stress can worsen the symptoms of sinusitis by increasing inflammation, impairing immunity, and intensifying discomfort and tension in the muscles. Acquiring proficiency in stress mitigation methods can lessen the negative effects of stress on sinus health and enhance general well-being. The following are some methods for stress management that promote sinus health:

- Mindfulness Meditation: This technique, which helps lower tension and encourage relaxation, entails concentrating your attention on the current moment without passing judgment. Spending a few minutes a day on mindfulness meditation can help ease tension in the body, especially the muscles that surround the sinuses, and quiet the mind and reduce anxiety.

- Deep Breathing Exercises: Deep breathing techniques, such as belly breathing and diaphragmatic breathing, can help lower tension and trigger the body's relaxation response. Breathe slowly and deeply through your nose, letting your abdomen expand with each inhalation and constrict with each exhalation. Breathing deeply helps ease muscular tension, promote nasal drainage, and soothe the neurological system.

- Yoga: Yoga promotes strength, flexibility, and relaxation via the use of physical postures, breathwork, and mindfulness practices. Asanas like forward folds, twists, and inversions can ease sinus pressure, promote better circulation, and lessen congestion. Including yoga in your daily practice can assist nasal health and help manage stress.

- Progressive Muscle Relaxation: To encourage relaxation and lessen stress, progressive muscle relaxation is methodically tensing and releasing various bodily muscle groups. Work your way up to your head by tensing and relaxing each muscle group, beginning with your toes. Progressive muscular relaxation is useful for reducing tension in the muscles and fostering general relaxation.

- Stress-Reduction Activities: Take part in relaxing and unwinding activities, such as taking a warm bath, practicing aromatherapy, spending time in nature, or listening to relaxing music. To reduce stress and promote sinus health, choose relaxing and joyful activities to include in your weekly or daily schedule.

- Cognitive behavioral therapy, or CBT, is a therapeutic method that assists patients in recognizing and altering harmful thinking processes and behavior patterns that fuel tension and anxiety. You can enhance your general well-being and acquire coping skills and ways to handle stress more skillfully by working with a therapist skilled in cognitive behavioral therapy (CBT).

- Healthy Lifestyle Practices: Make sleep a priority, eat a balanced diet, drink enough water, and limit your intake of caffeine, alcohol, and nicotine. Maintaining your general well-being can help lower stress, boost immunity, and promote sinus health.

Exercise and Sinus Health

Exercise regularly is crucial for sinus health support and general health maintenance. Exercise enhances immune system performance, lowers inflammation, increases circulation, and encourages healthy nasal discharge. Here are some suggestions for adding physical activity to your schedule and ways that exercise might improve sinus health:

- Cardiovascular Exercise: Aerobic exercises that enhance nasal drainage and circulation include walking, running, cycling, swimming, and dancing. For optimal sinus health and general well-being, spend at least half an hour most days of the week doing moderate-intensity aerobic activity.

- Pilates and yoga: These low-impact training styles emphasize breathwork, flexibility, and strength. A few yoga postures and Pilates movements can aid with sinus and chest opening, posture correction, and relaxation. To improve sinus health and lower stress, include yoga or Pilates in your exercise regimen.

- Strength Training: Activities that increase muscular strength and enhance general fitness include weightlifting, resistance band exercises, and bodyweight exercises. Robust muscles facilitate appropriate alignment and posture, hence mitigating stress and strain in the surrounding sinus muscles.

- Breathing Exercises: Include breathing exercises in your workouts to increase oxygenation, stimulate sinus drainage, and strengthen your lungs. To promote sinus health and lower stress, do deep breathing exercises during warm-up, cool-down, or relaxation times.

- Outdoor Activities: Take part in physical pursuits like hiking, gardening, or sports while spending time outside. Sunlight and fresh air may improve mood, ease stress, and promote general health and well-being. Just be aware of outdoor irritants like pollen or air pollution, which can make some people's sinusitis symptoms worse.

- Listen to Your Body: Observe how exercise affects your body and modify your regimen accordingly. Try changing the amount, length, or style of exercise to better fit your requirements and preferences if you have nasal congestion or pain during or after.

- Remain Hydrated: To keep hydrated and promote healthy nasal drainage, drink lots of water before, during, and after activity. Make careful to frequently rehydrate yourself because dehydration can exacerbate nasal congestion and pain, especially during severe or extended activity sessions.

MEAL PREP AND PLANNING

Keeping a nutritious diet, saving time, and decreasing stress in your daily life are all important goals that may be accomplished via the use of meal preparation and planning tactics. You will be able to guarantee that you have alternatives that are both nutritious and delicious and accessible throughout the week if you plan your grocery shopping and prepare your meals in advance. In this all-encompassing book, we will discuss the advantages of meal preparation, the methods for cooking in large quantities, and the suggestions for effectively shopping for groceries.

Batch Cooking for Convenience

Preparing a large amount of food at once to divide out and enjoy over the week is known as batch cooking. When you're short on time, this method can help you prepare meals more quickly and efficiently while also assisting you in choosing healthier options. Here's how to add batch cooking to your daily meal preparation schedule:

- Pick Recipes Carefully: Opt for recipes that work well in large quantities, such as casseroles, soups, stews, and one-pot dishes. These recipes are easily doubled or tripled to make several meals, and the leftovers are frequently much more delicious.

- Invest in Storage Containers: To fit your batch-cooked meals, stock up on a range of premium storage containers in various sizes. Choose glass or BPA-free plastic containers, or reusable silicone bags that are dishwasher, freezer, and microwave-safe.

- Begin by organizing your menu: Set aside some time at the start of each week to schedule your meals and snacks. Think about what meals you'll divide out and prepare in bulk, along with any extra items you might need for salads, sides, or fresh ingredients.

- Prepare Items Effectively: To speed up the process of preparing meals, wash, cut, and prepare ingredients ahead of time. Prepare veggies, marinade meats, or prepare grains and legumes ahead of time so they may be quickly added to meals all week long on the weekends or during a less hectic time.

- Make Use of Slow Cookers and Instant Pots: These kitchen appliances are crucial for large-scale cooking since they let you prepare meals in advance and then forget about them while they cook. With the help of these gadgets, easily prepare big quantities of soups, stews, or shredded meats for meal prep.

- Portion Out Meals: Using your storage containers, divide your prepared meals into individual servings as soon as they are done. Mark containers with the contents and date so you can remember what's inside and when it was made.

- Freeze Extras: If you've prepared more food in bulk than you'll use in a week, save the excess in the freezer for another time. To make quick and easy dinners on busy days, divide leftovers into quantities that are suitable for a single serving and freeze them in freezer-safe containers or bags.

- Change Up the Foods: Vary up your weekly batch-cooked recipes to keep mealtimes engaging. To keep mealtimes interesting and make sure you're receiving a range of nutrients in your diet, try experimenting with new flavors, cuisines, and ingredients.

Grocery Shopping Tips

Effective grocery shopping is necessary for well-planned and prepared meals. You can maximize your grocery shop visits and make sure you have all you need for wholesome meals throughout the week by stocking up on necessities, adhering to a budget, and reducing food waste. Here are some pointers for shrewd supermarket shopping:

- Write a List: Based on the meals and snacks you have planned for the week, make a list of the things you need before you go to the grocery store. To make your shopping trip more efficient, group your list by categories (such as vegetables, dairy, and pantry items).

- Organize Your Meals: Make your grocery list based on the items in your meal plan. To determine which ingredients you currently have on hand and which ones you need to buy, check your pantry, refrigerator, and freezer.

- Shop the Periphery: In the majority of grocery shops, the areas closest to the entrance are where you'll find fresh vegetables, meats, dairy, and baked goods. Since these are typically healthier selections, concentrate on stocking your cart with whole, unprocessed foods from these categories.

- Examine the labels: When choosing packaged goods, spend some time reading the ingredient lists and nutrition labels. Select whole grain items whenever you can, and keep an eye out for goods with low levels of artificial chemicals, added sugars, and salt.

- Invest in Bulk: By buying pantry essentials like grains, legumes, nuts, seeds, and dried fruits in large quantities, you can save costs and packaging waste. To keep bulk things at home, think about investing in reusable jars or containers.

- Keep to Your Budget: Before your food shopping excursion, decide on a spending limit and try your best to stay within it. Focus on your list and give necessities a higher priority than non-essentials to avoid making impulsive purchases.

- Reduce Food Waste: To reduce food waste, properly plan your meals and portion amounts. To further extend your grocery budget, go for products that are adaptable and can be used in several dishes. You may also plan to use leftovers in future meals.

- Shop Seasonally: Make the most of the fresher, more delicious, and more reasonably priced fruit that is in season. To acquire access to locally grown fruits and vegetables, visit farmers' markets or sign up for a community-supported agriculture (CSA) program.

- Think About Online Shopping: If you're short on time or would rather avoid crowded markets, you might want to look into meal delivery kits or online grocery shopping services. A lot of stores provide easy ways to purchase groceries online and have them delivered right to your house.

- Keep It Organized: To make grocery shopping simpler and more effective, keep your meal plan, recipes, and grocery list arranged in either paper or digital form. To make the process go more quickly, think about utilizing printable templates or meal-planning applications.

CONCLUSION

If you take the appropriate approach, it is possible to get relief from the symptoms of sinusitis and enhance your overall quality of life. Sinusitis may be a difficult condition to treat. Throughout the entirety of this book, we have discussed a variety of facets of sinusitis, including its causes, symptoms, treatment choices, nutritional concerns, lifestyle modifications, and tactics for meal planning. As we come to a close, let's review the most important issues that were discussed in this book and talk about strategies to go forward and live a healthy life while having sinusitis.

Looking Ahead: Living Well with Sinusitis

When you have sinusitis, you need to take continuous care of your health and well-being. Even if there could be obstacles in your path, you also have the chance to take charge of your symptoms and lead a happy life. Here are some important things to think about going forward:

- Remain Up to Date: Maintain your education on the treatment of sinusitis. Keep abreast of the most recent findings, available therapies, and practical lifestyle choices to ensure successful disease management.

- Interact with Your Medical Team: Be in constant contact with your healthcare provider(s) on your symptoms, your treatment regimen, and any queries or worries you may have. Together, come up with a thorough plan for treating your sinusitis.

- Emphasis on Prevention: Take precautions to avoid recognized triggers, such as allergens, pollutants, and respiratory infections, to prevent flare-ups of sinusitis. Reduce the likelihood of repeated sinusitis episodes by maintaining proper cleanliness, drinking enough water, and adhering to your treatment plan religiously.

- Pay Attention to Your Body: Keep an eye on how your body reacts to various foods, activities, and surroundings. Adapt your treatment plan, nutrition, and lifestyle choices as necessary to your unique symptoms and experiences.

- Make self-care a priority. Set aside time for things that will help you relax, cope with stress, and feel better overall. Take part in the things that make you happy and fulfilled, such as practicing mindfulness, having hobbies, or spending time with close ones.

- Remain upbeat: Keep an optimistic attitude and concentrate on the things under your control. Even though having sinusitis might be difficult, it's still vital to be proactive and upbeat about taking care of your health and live life to the fullest.

To sum up, managing sinusitis effectively necessitates a comprehensive strategy that takes into account nutritional, behavioral, and medical aspects. You may successfully manage your symptoms, lessen the frequency of flare-ups, and enhance your general quality of life by adopting healthy behaviors, being educated, and keeping an optimistic outlook. Keep in mind that you are not traveling alone and that there are resources available to assist you in overcoming the difficulties associated with having sinusitis.